GRANNY TELLS HER STORY, AND YOU WON'T BELIEVE IT!

BY HILDA TOSH

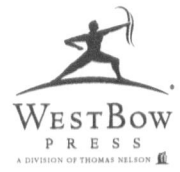

WestBow
PRESS

A DIVISION OF THOMAS NELSON

WestBow Press books may be ordered through booksellers or by contacting:

WestBow Press
A Division of Thomas Nelson
1663 Liberty Drive
Bloomington, IN 47403
www.westbowpress.com
1-(866) 928-1240

ISBN: 978-1-4497-9864-2 (sc)
ISBN: 978-1-4497-9865-9 (e)

Library of Congress Control Number: 2013910894

Scripture taken from the King James Version of the Bible.

Printed in the United States of America.

WestBow Press rev. date: 6/20/2013

TABLE OF CONTENTS

INTRODUCTION

HI MY NAME IS HILDA TOSH, and this is my story. I know that some of what I am going to share will be hard to believe and some will be very believable. Now at the age of 84 looking back on my journey of life I even find some of it hard to believe. Some of what I will share will make you laugh and some may make you cry, but, it is my hope and prayer that you will look at it as a miracle. I say that because I know for sure that if God had not had His hand on me from the time I was born, I would not be telling you my story.

You may ask me why at my age I would want to tell it all. The reasons are many. First; I want to give glory to my Father God for all the mercy and grace He has given me. Second; I have grandchildren and family that I have never met, and I want to give them something that will help them to know me and understand that even though I never got to meet them in this life I love them and pray for them. Last of all; I would like people to understand that no matter what circumstances they may find themselves in God is always there for them.

My life has been full and enriched with many friends along the way. I have traveled and seen almost every state in the union. I have had much and I have had little in the way of worldly possessions, but nothing can compare with the joy I have had in knowing Jesus as my Lord and Savior. I am grateful to have my story to tell and even more grateful to know that I have a home waiting for me in heaven when it's my time to leave this world.

Until that day comes I have much to look forward to. My Father knows that I love adventure and working in His kingdom, so as my life continues I just may have to write a sequel to this book, and you probably won't believe that either.

WHERE IT STARTED

I WAS BORN IN VERMONT OCTOBER 29, 1928 to Fred and Bertha Utter. I had a total of four brothers and three sisters who lived and two siblings that passed shortly after birth. I don't remember them or their gender because they were born before I was. My surviving siblings' names were Charles, Cornelia, Lillian, Kenneth, Norman, Millard and Doris.

Times were very different in the day that we all grew up in rural Vermont. By the time I was old enough to remember stuff Charles, Cornelia and Lillian were already grown and had moved away. Kids usually moved out on their own as soon as they were able to get jobs and find a way to support themselves.

When I was about eight years old we lived on a dairy farm where my brother Kenneth and I milked cows before and after school. We had to milk to have money for the family to live on. The milk provided money to buy supplies for our family.

One of my most vivid memories of living on the dairy farm was of the day my younger brother Millard almost got burned to death in the old milking barn. I remember seeing smoke coming from inside the barn. We could hear Millard inside crying but could not get inside because the barn door was locked. We yelled like crazy for mama and she came and got

Millard out of the barn. Dad had locked him in an old truck in the barn and set it on fire. I never knew what Millard did to make dad so mad. It never really took much it seemed. My dad was not a drinking man, but he sure was mean as a snake. He was very harsh. I do not remember anything kind he ever said to us kids. I remember always being on his bad side. From the time I can remember, I stayed in trouble with him. I hated the way he treated my mother and us kids so I was always back talking him. Of course this never made anything better. The scars I carry on my legs and back to this day remind me of that.

My mom, on the other hand, was a very mild natured person. She loved us kids and would try her best to keep us in line. My mother worked very hard and kept the family going the best she could. I can only guess what she put up with. Times were so hard back then it was rare for a woman, especially one with kids, to walk away from her husband and start over. Most of the time they just stayed till they died, and that's just what mama did.

Not long after the episode with Millard our family left the farm and moved to Essex Junction, Vermont in Chittenden County. This did not make our lives any better, but our chores changed from milking cows to chopping wood and hunting food.

The winters were very harsh where we lived. I can remember the snow blowing in through the cracks in the walls of our bedroom. Life was a rollercoaster of survival. We were very poor and had to supplement our food supply with whatever we could kill. I can remember eating bear and just about any other wild animal that we could find. Kids grow up very fast when they live in an atmosphere of self preservation.

From the time we were old enough to go outside by ourselves we were doing chores. We always tried to find something to amuse ourselves. We sometimes got into some pretty good jams by pulling our pranks. Being the dare devil that I was, I usually found some mischief to get into.

I guess I was born with a stubborn streak. From the time I can remember I hated being told what to do. I was "Little Miss Independent". I hated my big brother Kenneth telling me what to do. He just seemed to love bossing me around, but he also watched out after me so I didn't get the life beat out of me by dad. I can look back now and realize that he probably saved my life by running interference between me and dad.

Once when Kenneth and I were going across a field where some cows were, I thought it would be funny to mess with the bull. I aggravated that bull until he decided to chase us. Here we went screaming to the top of our lungs and running as fast as our legs would go. I was much smaller than Kenneth so I managed to scoot under the fence but he had to run to a nearby tree and climb up to a safe limb. I laughed at him until he was mad enough to hurt me, but since he was in the tree there wasn't much he could do. Kenneth kept telling me to go get dad, but I wasn't about to. Finally dad heard him yelling and came got him down from the tree. Luckily for me Kenneth was the one who got into trouble for that stunt.

I remember one day when Kenneth and I were out cutting wood. All we had to cut it with was a cross cut saw and an ax. I would get on one side of the log and Kenneth would get on the other. He loved to torment me with that saw. I would pull one side and he would pull it back and if we worked together we would get the job done. Needless to say that usually ended with a fight. Kenneth loved to pull back on the saw so that when I went to pull it through to cut it made it very difficult. He really thought it was funny to aggravate me. That day he really got on my one nerve.

After we cut the log we began splitting the smaller pieces into fire wood. That Kenneth just kept on bugging me. I was trying to use the ax and make the pieces small enough to use in the stove. I was just chopping away, and Kenneth began daring me to chop off his finger. He would put it down on the chopping block and grab it back just to dare me. Well finally I had enough, and he put his finger on the block and down came the ax and off came his finger from the knuckle down. He couldn't believe I did it even though he dared me. We both thought dad would kill me for doing it. We both knew how dad loved to use his chain on us. Somehow though Kenneth was able to handle dad enough I was spared a beating. It seems strange now to remember how Kenneth and I fought as kids, but he always seemed to be looking out for me.

An enjoyable memory I have with Kenneth is our dancing outings. Mom would allow me and him to sneak off and go into town to the Saturday night dance. I think my mom must have had a soft spot for me and Kenneth because of how we were treated. She would do what she could get away with to make our lives a little easier.

People from all over would come, and it was fun to watch the band play and people laugh and have a good time. It was an escape from the hard economic times everyone was having. Mom made us be careful to make sure dad did not find out, and this made it even more fun for us. It was our secret fun life so to speak. Kenneth and I became the bell of the ball when we would dance. We would skirt around the dance floor and have a ball. We would win trophies for our dance moves. Of course we would have to hide them so dad would not find them, but that was part of the fun for us. This will always be one of my fondest memories of my brother.

I also remember helping my mom empty wash water. Doing laundry in those days consisted of drawing water from the well and using wash pots to heat it. My mother was carrying my baby sister and was due anytime. She had just finished doing the laundry and was worn out when she ask me to help her empty the wash tubs, and my dad threw a fit. I still helped her knowing I would be in trouble with dad. Sure enough he used the chain on my back. I think he enjoyed making my mother work like a slave.

Not long after my mother had my little sister she became very ill. I still don't know what was wrong with her. She just seemed to fade away. Dad would not answer any questions about her illness. I was eleven when she died. I remember some men coming to the house and carrying her down the stairs wrapped in a quilt taking her to the hospital, but she never came home. It was a sad time for us kids because she was the only kind thing we had in our lives. We were never allowed to know anything else about her. We weren't allowed to talk to him about her. Dad just pretended she was never there.

I know that I was natured to be ornery, but I think the coldness of our family upbringing just made me bitter. I think us kids learned how to survive and did what we could to make it day to day. After mom died it just seemed to become more than I could handle. I was very angry by this time and hated my dad more than anything.

To make it worse, he remarried almost immediately after mom died. My stepmother was very harsh like my dad. I can only guess, but I assume she had decided to line us kids out.

She had seven kids of her own. It was a disaster from the start. There was no way she was going to take my mother's place in my eyes. At twelve years old I had developed an attitude of "enough is enough".

One morning as we were getting ready for school I heard my little sister give out a terrible scream. I ran up the stairs to find that my stepmother had slapped my sister so hard that it left a hand print across her face. Before I knew it I had grabbed the broom and knocked my stepmother down the stairs. She was hurt but not enough to keep her from threatening us with dad. My brother Kenneth knew that dad would beat me to death with the chain when he got home, so he had me pack a bag, and at the age of twelve my fourteen year old brother took me to the train station and we hopped a box car heading for Boston to my older sisters. I literally ran for my life.

As I left home for good that day, I couldn't help but worry about my little brothers and sister. I didn't know what would become of them, but at twelve years of age and scared out of your mind I had no choice but to run. When Kenneth and I hopped the train in Burlington and headed to Boston MA. to my sister Cornelia's house, I never looked back. I knew that my life was about to change, and I could only hope for the better.

Cornelia was married to Louie Demarais, and they had one daughter named Janice. She was much older than I was and so I really did not know her, but thank God she took me in and I lived with her until I married when I was sixteen. Kenneth chose to go back and face dad. I know it was rough for him, but I also know he looked after Norman, Millard and Doris. For that I am grateful.

I never went back home until my dad died. After I received

the call I knew I had to go see for myself that he was really dead. He had been working as a school janitor and was found passed away in the basement of the school. I know it sounds hard now to some, but all I knew was hate from him, and so I grew up hating him. In time I did overcome that hate and came to realize that as Christ had healed me from the pain of my past, I must forgive also. Forgiveness is not an easy thing to do for anyone, but when you finally can reach that place where you let go of the hurt and pain, the peace you receive is worth the journey.

How sad it is that today, seventy-two years later, these kinds of stories are repeated every day. Child abuse and neglect are common occurrences. Kids are left to fend for themselves and are abused by alcoholic or drug addicted parents who really don't care about what happens to them. Children go hungry so parents can feed their addictions. This young generation for the most part is an angry one. Their pain is very real. I know that it is the same today as it was for me at age twelve. Only God can heal the pain of an ugly childhood. It took me a lot of years to get to that point, but thank God I met Jesus one day and although I still have the scars on my outward body, my inward man is healed from my childhood pain.

NEW BEGINNING
AT TWELVE

When Kenneth and I hopped that box car in Burlington, Vermont headed to my sisters in Boston, Massachusetts I knew I would never go back home. I never looked back. The next time I went back was to go to my dad's funeral. I went for only one reason and that was to make sure he was dead. I would not have believed it unless I saw him for myself. I guess I felt like the nightmares of my childhood would die with him but they didn't.

I did not realize it at the time, but my little sister Doris never forgave me for leaving her behind. I was only twelve and she was two. I couldn't have taken care of her at the time because I was just a kid myself. Taking her would have given him a reason to follow me and I feared that.

I never knew the depth of the pain she suffered at the hands of my dad and stepmother. It was not until I went back to Vermont to visit my family in 2009 that she shared some of her pain with me. The details of her time with dad were always overshadowed by unforgivness and bitterness. My sister had had a lovely man as a husband and two children, but as she shared with me about her feelings toward me I knew that she had many scars and a lifetime of regrets she had never dealt with.

It is strange that the pains we hold on to from past hurts haunt us for a lifetime if we don't deal with them and let go of the grudges and bitterness. Most of the time we don't realize that childhood pain can ruin any future happiness we may be blessed with if we always are looking back.

The healing that Jesus brought to us on the cross was more than physical. Sometimes people need an emotional healing more than a physical one. The truth is that if we hold on to old hurts and childhood pain it will keep us from ever being truly happy. Jesus died so that we could have healing for the whole man, that includes the spirit, soul (mind-will-emotions), and the physical body.

I have seen people go to the grave with bitterness and unforgivness, and what good did it do them or anyone else? Most people I have known would change their lives in some way if they could go back in time. Since we are not afforded that privilege, we just have to lay it at Jesus' feet and take up our lives and follow after Him to have a better future than what the past gave us.

My hope and prayer is that my sister will make peace with her past and have some peace of mind before she goes to meet the Lord.

When Kenneth and I were in the box car headed to our sister's, our emotions were running high. Not knowing what to expect when we got there and knowing that I could not go back to dads. It seemed like forever riding in the dark car, but we finally stopped in the depot. When the conductor found us hiding in the car, he was surprised to find two kids. He immediately inquired of us where we thought we were going. Kenneth would not speak up and kept punching me to talk. Finally I told him that we were going to our sister's house. He got the phone number from us and called her. Needless to say she was very surprised to find out that we were there. She did come, however, and took us to her house. After a few days Kenneth went back home to dad, but I stayed with Connie.

Connie and her husband, Louie, were very good to me. I know they did not really know what to do with me at first, but we soon settled into a family environment and I helped them with their young daughter, Janice. I didn't know what to expect when I first arrived, I only knew that I had to get away from dad. Connie understood all too well, and for that reason, I believe she was more than willing to help me get a new start in life.

I looked for work and found a job working in the ship yard. Boston was home to the US Navy fleet. The ships would come in for repairs or just so the sailors could have a little R&R. I always looked a little older than I really was, so lying about my age worked to get me the job. I told them I was sixteen when really I was only fourteen. My boss was ok with my working at a young age because almost everyone had to work in those days to eat and get by. He did however question me after I turned fifteen. When I confessed to my age he agreed to keep me on if I would not tell anyone else how young I was. I worked very hard and was careful to make a good hand so that I could stay with Connie. Wages were low but with Connie and Louie both working we made it pretty good. For the first time in my life, I felt worth something. I was always independent and head strong and in the situation I was in at such a young age, it did help me make it through some tough times.

Life pretty much settled into a routine for me. I would go to work and home to help Connie with Janice. Days passed and before I knew it I turned fifteen. I walked to work because I sure wasn't old enough to drive and couldn't afford a car anyway, but I was ok with that. I would walk past the ships that came into harbor and down through the local shops. I had a favorite restaurant I liked to stop in everyday.

One day as I was sitting in one of the booths a young good looking sailor came and sat down across from me and began talking to me. I thought he was so handsome in his uniform. We would talk about everything we could think of. He was good at conversation. His name was Johnny Calvert. His ship was in dry dock for repairs. It had suffered bomb damage, and he had to stay there while his ship was being fixed which gave us time to get to know each other. After the third time of meeting him in the café, he asked me to a movie. We hit it off very well. We gave each other someone to talk to. Johnny was from Alabama and was scheduled to be shipped back overseas when his ship was repaired.

The courtship was a brief one. When Johnny began talking about marriage, I wasn't sure I wanted to get married at such a young age. Johnny was the first boy I ever dated. It was a whole new ball game for me. He was so convincing and sure of himself. He made it all sound so wonderful.

He was twenty two, and I was about to turn sixteen. It took some convincing, but I began to feel like this was an opportunity for a new life. I had fallen for Johnny by this time and loved him enough to commit to marriage. I turned sixteen on October 29, 1945, and we were married November 5, 1945.

Soon after the wedding, his orders to return overseas came through. He decided to send me to Alabama to his parents to live while he finished his tour overseas. So I went on another adventure as a new bride. When I arrived at his parents' home in Alabama I found two loving people who took me in and took care of me until Johnny came home.

NEW BEGINNING
WITH JOHNNY

AFTER ABOUT SIX MONTHS, JOHNNY CAME home from the Navy. We bought a little farm in Crane Hill, Alabama. We farmed cotton and worked from sun up to sun down. There wasn't much time for anything else, so we just worked and took care of the farm. There were no special times that I can remember. Johnny and I both just worked and tried to make a go of the farm.

I had my first child, Kenneth, on April 9, 1947; about two years after Johnny came home. I was so excited to be a mom. I was determined that my children would have the kind of home I never had when I was growing up. Johnny loved Kenneth too and we just kept working and trying to keep the farm going. I would take Kenneth with me to the cotton fields and pull him behind me as I picked cotton. Life just passed by from day to day.

I really don't know why we sold our farm. Johnny kept all the business part of our marriage, so I never knew anything about the financial part. One day for whatever reason we sold the farm and moved to Fairfield, Alabama. I went to work in the local Burger King, and Johnny went to work in the steel factory. I had my second son, Steve, in 1952. I was very content being a mom. I loved the boys and worked hard to be a good mom.

It was very hard sometimes working and being a full time mom and wife. Johnny grew very discontent during those difficult times. I don't know if it was the fact that we had to give up the farm we worked so hard to keep or if it was just the disappointment of a failed dream. It got to the place that he was a very unhappy man. I could do nothing to please him. I felt like a failure and did not know why. I don't want to tell Johnny's story because I don't really know what his story was other than he changed and blamed me for our losses. People do that all the time when they need a scapegoat to blame. Perhaps I was a disappointment to him. I really don't know. If I couldn't figure it out then, I know there is no use trying to figure it out now.

Out of the clear blue one day when Kenneth was seven, Johnny came home from work and threw me out of the house. Even though things were bad between us, I didn't see that one coming. There was no forewarning, no threats beforehand of doing so, just bam and it happened. I found myself locked out. He kept the boys from me, and I was forced to sleep in my car and rely on friends to help me out. I tried to get back home, but Johnny would have none of it. Just a few days later, he moved into the house with a woman he worked with and took my little boys with him. Shortly thereafter, he filed for divorce and full custody of our boys.

I did manage to get a lawyer and face Johnny in court. When the time came to go to court, I was still unsettled with no place of my own to live. I did have a job and a car but no permanent place to live. Things were still in shock mode for me. I couldn't believe it all happened. One day I am a mom with children the next Johnny was asking the court to take them away from me. The judge was very sympathetic and understood my predicament. He made Johnny pay all the lawyer fees and court costs but because I was homeless with no way to provide a home for the kids he did allow Johnny to take the boys. I was also told that as soon as I could provide a stable home for the boys the judge would revisit my case and allow me to have the boys. I had to be able to provide shelter, food and care for the boys. I was given liberal visitation with the boys and was supposed to be able to see them and spend time with them while I worked on providing a home for them. There were no social services such as food stamps or shelter vouchers like they have today back when I was a young mother. Had there been and help available I would not have lost the boys. I had to start from scratch and try to overcome the tragedy of losing my children and rebuilding my life that had been ripped to shreds.

My world collapsed the day I walked out of that court room. I was alone and lost in my despair. I had no family to turn to and only had my love for the boys to encourage me to pick up the pieces and rebuild my broken heart.

For weeks I tried to see the boys. Each and every time I tried Johnny denied my request. I showed up at the house he was living with his girl friend and was always turned away. He blocked every effort I made to see my children. He refused to obey the court order for my visitations, and having no way to hire a lawyer to go back to court, I finally fell prey to his denial of my right to visit my sons. Shortly after our divorce was final, Johnny married his girlfriend and completely cut me out of any contact with the boys.

After all my efforts to be part of their lives failed, I took courage and decided to rebuild my life so I could return and take Johnny back to court for the boys. This I knew would take time, but I was willing to do what I could to make it happen.

It got so unbearable for me to be close to the boys and not be able to see them that I decided to move to Tyler, Texas. I was determined to work hard and make a way to be a mom again to the boys. With new determination I set out on what would become another leg in the journey of my life.

THEN THERE WAS JAMES

W HEN A PERSON WRITES THEIR MEMOIRS, they have to look back into their past and remember why certain events were memorable. As they write those events, it will always bring them to reflect on those events. In doing so, we may ask ourselves what we may have done differently if we could change the past. Unfortunately, we are never afforded that privilege. Reflecting on the past events of our lives will also give us a determination to make changes for our future. We might say to ourselves, "I will never do that again", but often we do make the same unwise choices again, especially when we choose to make those decisions without God's wisdom.

I have to remember, when looking back, that at this time of my life I did not know God. I know now that He knew me and was always there protecting me and helping me until I would accept Him and give my life to Him. I, however, did not have knowledge of Him at this stage of my life. I never prayed about anything. Like most young girls, I depended on my own choices to make things happen for me. As you continue reading my memoirs, you can see how that worked out for me.

I went back to work at Burger King in Tyler and began to get my life together. It was difficult to start over again, but I felt

I had a good reason to press on. The boys I left behind were the inspiration that kept me going during those lonely days. I dreamed of the day I could return and be able to hold them in my arms again. They were the only good thing I had been able to obtain in my young life, and I felt lost and alone without them.

One day a young man by the name of James Carnes came into the Burger King and I guess you might say he swept my heart away. He was good looking and very smooth talking. I still wasn't in a hurry to remarry but finally after about a year of being by myself I married James.

I know women sometimes live in fantasy worlds, but I think I fell hook line and sinker into what I will call the James world. I was a young girl in love with a world of dreams. My passion in life was to settle down and have a good marriage so that I could go back and get my children. I had lived on the words the judge told me about coming back to get them when I could provide a safe place for them. James knew all about my losing my children and was very supportive of us becoming a family; for a while anyway.

I kept working at Burger King and trying to get my life together. Then little by little my dream faded away. I had put my faith in James to be the husband that would help me build a life for my boys but in actuality he never intended to help me get my children back. He was good at making promises but failed to follow through on any of them.

I guess looking back I just gave up on ever being stable enough to go back and get my boys. By this time, Johnny and his new wife had settled in and with time passing and me not being allowed to see them at all, right or wrong on my part I figured they were probably better off without me in their lives. My life was such an unhappy mess, and I didn't have anything to offer them. I kept sending birthday cards and Christmas cards and presents, but I honestly don't know if they ever got any of them.

Without trying to make any excuses for my bad choices, I would like to say something here. Young girl, especially those who have not had any role models of good parents, really don't know how to make good choices. We grow up determined to make better choices with our lives than our parents did, but too many times we go down the same path they did. Unhealthy parents raise unhealthy children. Society expects us to make perfect, wonderful choices for our futures when the truth is; *we don't know how to make those choices!* I know that even good parents have children who make bad life choices, but the odds are much smaller for those who have had parents with good parenting skills. Children who are raised in loving families know that when they mess up they are still loved. That love usually gives the child the courage to make changes in their choices. You know if you think about it there is no difference between the boys or girls here. How a child is raised makes the difference in what kind of adult they become.

I will share more in later chapters about how I came to serve God, but I will add here that I am grateful that even though it took me years and years to come to see my need for a Heavenly Father, I know He was there all the time loving me and wanting me to make better choices, but I just wasn't ready to listen to Him at this point of my life. Had I been I am sure it would have saved me years of heartache and pain. Thank God for His patience towards me until He could finally make me see my need for Him.

My dream of retrieving my children faded. I just lived from

day to day. I vowed to never have any more children. I was determined not to have my heart broken again in that way. I decided that if I couldn't be a mother to my boys, I would not be a mother to any more kids. I hardened my heart to my marriage and I guess I quit trying to make it happen so to speak. That may have caused some of the discord with James, I don't know. We humans just have a way of turning off our emotions so that we can't feel the pain that is deep inside. There are always two sides so I can onlyguess that possibly I turned James off from ever being a family with me. Perhaps my desire to get my children back drew me to him in the first place. My motives may have been wrong in wanting to get married. I guess a person can second guess themselves over and over when they look back over their lives. is HHH

After a couple of years of marriage, James decided to move us to California. We moved to Gardenia. I think he wanted to have a fresh start, but it seemed to only make our relationship more distant. I got a job in the casinos. I played poker for the house. James just worked here and there and even though he was not a drinker, he sure loved to chase women. I resolved myself to tolerate his behavior because I really didn't have any personal ambition for my life during this time. We didn't fight much because I reconciled myself to the way he was. He was happy with this arrangement. It gave him the security to have other women without making any commitment to them. So he played his games, and I didn't bother with it. You might say life went on and time passed.

James and my relationship went on for about four more years. Neither one of us were happy even though we didn't argue much. We tolerated each other. One day he just ran off with one of his girlfriends. I think he knew I didn't care. I never tried to get him to come back, and he never asked. I was perfectly happy in my misery.

I was never very good at hiding my feelings so I imagine I conveyed my disappointment in James straight to his heart at times. I think he felt he couldn't make me happy with anything he did, and I don't think he could have. My dream of becoming stable and having my children back was gone, and I blamed James for that. Broken dreams and failed expectations are a sure destruction for marriage, especially one that is built only on those dreams and expectations. I knew nothing about forgiveness at this stage of my life, so I held it all in and carried the burden in my heart. My broken heart made me unhappy, cold and bitter. I am grateful that I can look back now and realize that I was wrong to blame James. My unhappiness was in me and not because of him. I am sorry that he had to suffer through this miserable time of my life with me, but actually he just seemed to fill his time with women and having a good time. I guess that is the way he dealt with his own pain. Needless to say, neither of us were winners in the relationship area.

I can only imagine my emotional state at this time, but I must have been a very depressed person because I just wanted my life to end. Depression is a cruel enemy. It makes you not care about yourself or anyone else. I really felt like I had no reason to go on with my life. Everything I had tried to accomplish with my life had failed. I had lost the two loves of my life when my boys were taken away from me and could not seem to find a reason to go on. I focused on my job and managed to get up every day but time meant nothing to me. Days went into weeks and weeks into years.

One day while driving down Highway 101 from Long Beach to San Diego, I decided to drive off one of the cliff roads. The highway is winding and at that time had no guard rails that kept cars that ran off the road from plunging off the side of the cliffs. As I got up the courage and was headed toward a curve determined to end it all, my car stalled and died. I could not get it to start for anything. As I was getting more aggravated, I heard a voice speak to me to "GO HOME". I was completely stunned but as you would think I ignored it. I kept trying to start my car with more determination to end it all. The frustration level was very high by now. The voice came again even with more volume. I was quite taken back by this time and had to sit and think about it. I didn't know the Lord at this time in my life, so you can imagine my fear at hearing a strange voice when no one was around. After thinking about it for a while, I decided to just go home. Even my attempts to end it all were failing, or so I thought. When I made up my mind to go home, to my surprise my car started. I was quite shaken after the incident. I made up my mind after that to settle in and just work and live my life day to day.

I believe we all have guardian angels and that day mine was really looking out for me. I'm grateful to this day for the mercy God showed me. A few years later as He began making Himself real to me, I could understand why God spared my life that day on Highway 101.

THEN THERE
WAS LEE

AFTER MY DIVORCE FROM JAMES I quit my job in the casinos and went to work in a sewing factory. The job was fine and less stressful. I made friends easily and soon settled in my "new" single life.

I had a neighbor friend that I worked with, and she introduced me to her cousin Lee Tosh. I had been divorced about six months and was not looking for another relationship with a man, but Lee was very handsome and I found myself in love again. Lee and I had only dated for a few months and he asked me to marry him. We went to Las Vages and got married and once again I started a new life. We settled in our new lives, and things went well for a couple of years. We continued to live in Gardenia where Lee drove a truck for Mayflower, and I continued to work in the sewing factory.

After about two years we decided to sell our house and move to Missouri. I had moved so much in my life it just seemed like another adventure to me. I also knew that if it made Lee happy then I would be happy. I went to work in Ironington, and Lee continued to drive for Mayflower Trucking. We settled down and bought a house. It seemed like it was going to work out this time for me. Little did I know what God had in store!

Lee was gone most of the time, but I busied myself with work and home. I was happy enough but found myself getting sick. I was not the kind of person to be sickly, but this seemed serious. After going to the doctor, I found out that I had throat cancer. It was in the late stages, and I was given only a few months to live. Needless to say, my world came crashing in on me again. I did not know which way to turn. There was not all the Chemotherapy treatments and options for recovery in those days as there are today. It was pretty much a death sentence.

Lee didn't take the news very well and withdrew from me as much as possible. I know now that it was his way of dealing with it. His truck driving job gave him a way to escape facing the truth about my cancer. I dealt with it as best as I could, but I sure was glad that as time went on I realized God had a plan all along.

One of my co-workers invited me to come along with her to church. I was not a church going person and the closest to any experience with a supernatural force was the voice that spoke to me on Highway 101 when I tried to kill myself. That was spooky enough, so I was not sure about the church thing. As I contemplated the invitation I had only one thought that kept going on in my mind and that was I had nothing to lose by going. So I finally gave in and went with her to church.

The church was Pentecostal, and I had heard some weird stuff about Pentecostals. Back in those days they were called "Holy Rollers", and I did not want any of them rolling over me. On the other hand I was dying anyway so knowing I had nothing to lose I went.

On my first visit to church with my friend, I was sitting on the back row and the pastor began operating in the Holy

Spirit with the gift of knowledge and called me out to come to the front to be prayed for. I slowly walked to the front not knowing what would take place, but I knew I had nothing to lose by going up for prayer. As the pastor began to pray for me, he looked straight at me and said, "You have cancer". I didn't know anything about the gifts of the Spirit and how God used them so I was shocked to say the least, but I knew he spoke truth to me. I had not told a single person about my condition, so I knew it must have been the Lord who showed him my situation. He told me that the Lord was going to heal me of the cancer, and he laid his hands on me and prayed. Immediately as he prayed the tumor in my throat began leaving. It took two times of his laying hands on me, but the cancer left my body. I was completely healed! After that the doctors found no trace of the tumor.

My faith seemed to grow by leaps and bounds after my healing. I had such an intimate loving experience with Jesus that I fell completely in love with Him. It was such a special relationship He began building in me, I felt truly loved for the first time in my life. Those of you who have experienced God's touch in such an awesome way know you are never the same. Your world rocks from the realization of being touched by such a loving Father. Not knowing where this journey would take me, I committed myself to Jesus and decided to follow Him. My choices in life had not proved to bring the happiness I so deeply desired so giving Jesus a chance seemed the right thing to do. I have never looked back or even wanted to go back to anything since that day. The love He filled my heart with eased all the ache the years of my past had caused. I finally had peace.

Lee did go to church some with me at first. He couldn't deny the miracle I had received in my body but somehow he just couldn't commit his life to Jesus. He struggled with going to church. My new found religion was overwhelming to him so he stayed gone on his truck as much as he possibly could. I was so caught up in my new life as a Christian that I really did not have time to beg him to come home and go to church. I was determined to build my relationship with Jesus, so I let a lot of things Lee did just fade in the distance.

As time went on, weeks turned into months and months into years, and my whole focus became the church. Before I knew it two years had gone by, and I couldn't have been happier. Things were not really that good between me and Lee, but I was still shocked to find out that he had a girlfriend on the side. He was gone on the road driving his truck most of the time, and I just worked and went to church. I guess I just never noticed how we had grown apart. We just had separate lives and were not involved enough with each other to see the hand writing on the wall. The hurt this time at being betrayed was different than before. I was hurt and disappointed that I had another failed marriage, but the love of God growing in my heart every day made this time a lot easier to accept. We divorced and he left town with his girlfriend, and we both moved on with our lives.

I had a nice home and a good car to drive and felt so blessed this go around not having to start over again from scratch. I decided that I would only be married to God and forget about ever trying to marry again. I know there are good Christian men out there but I decided I would not trade the peace I now had in my life to risk another failure in that department. I made that commitment to God and to this day have kept it.

Women are strange creatures sometimes. We dream and fantasize about perfect relationships and how our ideal person will come along to share our lives. Sometimes our greatest disappointments come from shattered dreams. Unless God is involved in our choice of a mate we never know what we will get when we choose out of the lust of the flesh. When you're young and foolish and don't have God involved in the life choices you make you are just bound for failure and disappointment. I found that out all too well.

You might say the above statement is just one an 84 year old lady is making and doesn't apply to me. Check yourself and see how your personal relationships are going. How many times have you been hurt or let down because someone you chose to share your intimate feelings with has disappointed you. Whether you are 84 or 14, when you choose to have a relationship with someone based on any other ingredient than God, it is a bad choice. You can have many casual friends, but close relationships you share your personal life with should have God involved in them.

It is because of those 84 years of experience and three failed marriages I can make an honest assessment of how to make better choices. Unfortunately, it is the same for every generation. We fail to learn from those who have "been there done that" so to speak. The reason for failed relationships is the same today as it was when I was a young girl. We make choices based on emotional feelings, fantasies, outward appearances, or financial status instead of prayer. If it is meant for a Christian girl or boy to marry, God has a mate prepared for them. If we could ever learn to wait on God and let Him do the picking we would see less broken homes and parentless children. Believe me when I say there are just as many fatherless and motherless children in the church houses as there are in the world. God help us!!

AND THEN GOD SAID MOVE ON

I WAS VERY CONTENT TO LIVE MY life day to day serving God and working. I loved my little house and enjoyed the peace I had in my heart. Peace within is a very precious commodity, it took me a long time to find it, so I was going to hang on to it no matter what, or so I thought. I would have been content to spend the rest of my life right where I was, but God seemed to have other plans.

You know it is so strange the way we humans try to figure God out. We will profess our devout love and dedication to Him, but we usually don't really mean it. The first time God messes with our little plans we get bent out of shape. We usually pray for His will to be done in our lives then go our way expecting things to go according to our plan.

I had spent all my time since Lee and I divorced dedicating myself to learning all I could about my Savior. I had fallen so in love with Jesus that I didn't want to be bothered with much of anything else. He gave me not only a sense of security for my life on this earth but a security of an eternal life in Heaven. I had been healed of cancer and was finding a new lease on life, or so I thought. I can only tell you that if you pray for the Lord to have His way in your life no matter what; you better mean it.

One April morning in 1973 I had come home from work, and as usual I was sitting on my porch swing reading my Bible and praying. The Holy Spirit spoke to me very gently and said, "Go to Bismarck, Arkansas". Well by this time of my spiritual growth I had learned to hear the voice of God but somehow I didn't want to believe that He was talking to me. I argued with the voice and got really angry, but He said again to me, "Go to Bismarck, Arkansas".

I said, "Ok God, I will call the capital of Arkansas to see if Bismarck even exists". I was so distraught by this time I was furious with God. I made the call and a sweet voice on the other end said, "Oh yes ma'am it's between Hot Springs and Arkadelphia, Arkansas. I was so mad at that lady. I couldn't believe it even existed, but once I knew it did, I had to be convinced I was really hearing from God.

Now I told you how much I loved my little house. Well, I wasn't about to give up my precious house too easily. Even though it was just a rental, it had become my sanctuary. I had peace of mind and contentment just living alone and filling my life with the presence of the Lord. I just didn't want to let go of that.

I really put a fleece before the Lord. I told God that if it was His will for me to go to a place I never heard of called Bismarck, Arkansas that I wanted my stuff all sold and everything settled quickly. Once I made that demand on God it was like a whirlwind hit my life. After two days of yard sale; I didn't even have a fork left to call my own. I had nothing left but my car, clothes, and a few dollars after I paid all my debts. I didn't even have a spare tire for my car!

As the time drew closer for me to leave and strike out to only God knew where, I grew exceedingly bitter. I let the anger I had and also the disappointment in God for asking such a thing of me to really get to me. I was totally under the influence of my bitterness as I headed out for a place I had never heard of, to find what I did not know. I was obedient to God in going, but my heart was not right in my submission to His will.

I know the Bible tells the story of Abraham and his obedience to God's voice when he was told to take his belongings and strike out to a place he did not know and blindly follow the leading of the Spirit of God. We look at this story as a great leap of faith, and we know the Bible calls Abraham the father of our faith. I can't help but believe though, that Abraham was full of mixed emotions as he began his journey. If you study the Word of God you see that Abraham did get into several confrontations with God along the way, and he managed to get into trouble too. He lied about his wife being his sister instead of his wife and got the king into trouble with God (Genesis 20:1-5). Now don't think I am comparing myself to Abraham other than the fact I had to pull up and move to a new place I didn't know just like he did. I would love to sit down with Abraham and ask him how he handled it emotionally. I would hope he did a better job than I did because I was a very angry, bitter person by the time I landed in Bismarck, Arkansas.

As I pulled into the little town of Bismarck, I noticed a small post office on the corner where two highways met. I went inside and asked if I had any mail. The postman of course told me no. How could I have mail? No one knew an address to send me mail, and I didn't know anyone in the area. I just figured God had got me there with seven dollars in my pocket and no place to stay or even direction as to what to do next.

As I sat in my car and mulled over the past few day's events, I told God that He had brought me here and He needed to tell me what I was to do next. I am surprised that I even heard Him through the emotional state of mind I was in, but I did hear Him tell me to go west on the highway and I would find a church to go to. I drove a little ways and didn't see anything, so I told God what I thought about that. He just patiently told me to keep going. I wish I could say I was happy when I saw the little church just ahead down the highway, but I wasn't at all pleased. I parked my car and went inside.

I would like to say that serving God is the easiest and most wonderful thing a person could do. However true that is, it does come with a price. Most Christians I know think Jesus did it all when He died on the cross. He certainly did pay the price for me to have forgiveness of my sins and come into a relationship with Father God, but we as believers must make the choice to take up *our* cross and follow. Our cross is our life with all its good and bad. All the bad stuff I have done along with the good things I have done. I must also face the fact that most of the choices I made for my life had only brought me heartache and pain.

As I stated before, when I gave my heart to Jesus I fell madly in love with Him. His love for me engulfed me and gave me a peace I had not known up to that time. I had looked for love in human relationships and had become very hurt and bitter because of the disappointment in those unwise decisions. I think when I drove up to that church in Bismarck I felt overwhelmed with that disappointment. I had decided to follow Jesus to the ends of the earth. Believe me I felt like I was at the end of my earth. Little did I know the journey that lay before me! I was meeting destiny. This place out in the middle of nowhere was the place my Father God had chosen for me to have a new beginning in Him. I sure was not in any frame of mind at the time to understand the meaning of that, but as time went on and God healed my hurt and forgave my bitterness, I learned to call Bismarck my home.

As I walked into that little Assembly of God church, I was certainly not in any mood to be gracious to anyone. As the people greeted each other before service time I sure felt out of place. The pastor came over to shake my hand and very casually said to me, "Hello sis, the Lord sent you here didn't He?" I could have slapped him for that remark. I tried to be spiritually holy and not show him that my stress level was through the roof. I just grunted and settled in for the service. Afterward he again came up to me and remarked to me, "Hey sis, you are going to need a place to stay aren't you?" I just smarted off back to him that I would if I was going to stay in Bismarck. He must have realized I was not in a talking mood, but he was very kind anyway. He told me to go home with one of the sisters in the church, and she would help me. He was right and that church sister became a dear friend to me.

God does surround us with love, but sometimes we are just too fleshly to see it. When you are hurting and confused as to what God is doing in your life, it is easy to get into the flesh. I did not realize I had so many deep wounds in my spirit. God had brought me to a place I didn't know existed, and I was not a happy camper about it. I was disappointed in God for dragging me away from my first church family. It had been a place of safety for me. I had learned to know Jesus and had no intention of letting go of that security.

You know it's funny how we religious people view God. We can't see what He is doing *for* us when we only see what life has done *to* us. I didn't know at the time that it was Father's love that had brought me to this place. I didn't realize He was giving me a whole new beginning in Him. All I saw at the time was what I had given up. Bitterness eats the soul out of a person. Of all the hurts and disappointments I had been through in life, I must admit that at this point I felt that even God had hung me out to dry. How very wrong I was. You have heard that old idiom "you can't see the trees for the branches". Well I couldn't see any good for all the stuff in the way. I will always be grateful that Jesus covered me with His mercy and helped me through this difficult transition in my life. Looking back I can understand that He was bringing me out of my Egypt into my promise land.

The lovely sister who took me in and helped me told me of a sewing factory between Bismarck and Hot Springs that was a good place to work. I decided to go and apply for a job, but I had to lay down the law to God first. I told Him that if it was His will for me to work and stay here to not let the people at the sewing factory ask me one question. That was my requirement for getting a job and settling down. I arrived at the business and began walking in when a tall distinguished man came out the door and greeted me. He asked me if he could help me, and I just told him I needed a job. He just looked at me and told me to show up for work Monday morning. You can imagine how blown away I was that God answered my request in such a dramatic way.

The negative side to this tremendous blessing from God was that it closed the back door I kept open in case the opportunity arose for me to leave Bismarck. I guess the last and final straw that closed all doors for me leaving came about four months after I began working in the sewing factory. While at work one day, I received a call from a funeral home Gardenia. They informed me that Lee's new wife had shot him and killed him. Apparently, she had caught him cheating on her and simply killed him. The funeral home wanted me to pay for Lee's funeral, but I refused. It was bad enough that he divorced me for this new wife, but to ask me to pay for his funeral really was the last straw that closed all the doors for me to ever return to anything I felt like I left behind when I came to Arkansas.

I worked at the sewing factory for the next eight years, made many new friends, and finally began settling in and making a home for myself. I enjoyed the new church I found myself in until the pastor who had helped me resigned the church and moved on. I became uneasy in my spirit and after a time of prayer and seeking God, He led me to start attending the Bismarck Pentecostal Church. I made that my home church and have attended it ever since.

I became the Granny of the church. God began to fill my life with young people. I can't even remember how many young people I have mentored and taken under my wing. I filled my life with what I called my "kids". For the next thirty-five years, I watched them grow up and move on. Some are still serving God, some are not, and I'm sorry to say some have gone on to be with the Lord. But they were all my "kids". I think my Father God knew how much the hole in my heart for my own boys needed to be filled because He kept on sending kids my way. I was truly blessed to be a part of teaching them to follow Jesus. I tried to teach them that no matter what to hold on to Him. I believed if they could get that one fact settled in their spirit, no matter what came their way, they could have that truth as an anchor. Between work, church, and "kids" time came and went, and that was not a bad thing for me.

ANOTHER CHANGE

After eight years at the sewing factory another job came open. This one was at the State Park in our area. The job came with benefits and an opportunity for retirement. I took the housekeeping job and enjoyed working for the state for the next four years. I settled in and probably would have stayed for retirement until another chain of events changed my course once again.

My friend had opened a small sewing factory in another town close by and wanted me to come help her. I quit my job at the State park and went to work for her. I worked for her until 1986 when one of the ladies of my church, Ruth Baker, had a very serious car accident and was hurt very badly. They also had a daughter named Shryl who had Down's Syndrome and some heart issues. They needed someone to help take care of Ruth until she was on her feet again and see after Shryl.

I moved into the house with Frank and Ruth Baker and Shryl. I enjoyed helping out, and it was not long before Shryl and I became fast buddies. She was so pleasant to be around, and Frank and Ruth treated me like family. They actually became my family. For the first time since Johnny and I split up and I lost the boys I felt like I had a family. It was like pieces of a puzzle, and we all fit together. Frank built on to their house and gave me a little space of my own. We all shared the kitchen, but I had my own bedroom, living room, and bath. I have been with them ever since, and I must say I have been very content.

In 1997, Frank and Ruth bought some cottages close to Lake DeGray. Of all things they named them "Granny's Cottages". Thus the nickname *Granny* has become a legend. They made me the manager, and I'm still managing those cottages today. I guess going to live with the Bakers gave me my first permanent home. Their family became my family and because they loved to travel I am very blessed to have visited almost every state in the U.S. Frank always kept a camper or large van ready to go. Whenever they would take a notion, here we would go on a road trip. Shryl loves to travel, and we have had mountains of fun going down the highway on road trips.

God has been very good to me since He brought me to Bismarck. I can't imagine my life had I not obeyed Him and struck out in my old car to find a place I never heard of years ago. I have been able to have a loving family take me in and a church family that I dearly love. But the ache in my heart for my boys never went away.

I don't know how long ago perhaps ten years, I really got lonesome to find my boys. One of my dear friends in my church told me she would go on a road trip with me to see if we could find them. We prayed for success asked God to let us find them if it was His will, set the date, and off we went with only their last known address as our guide. Sure enough I was able to find my youngest son, Steve. He was very receptive to seeing me. We had a wonderful visit. Kenneth, my oldest, lived close by but was not interested in meeting me at that time. I didn't push and just enjoyed Steve and went home with a very grateful heart having seen my baby after so many years. I have been privileged to make a second trip to see Steve since then. We talk on the phone often, and I cherish hearing his voice. I hope to go again before long to see him.

I knew that Kenneth was unsure about seeing me because he felt I had just abandoned him when he was little. I understood those feelings and respected how he felt. I just prayed that one day he would find it in his heart to forgive me and allow me to meet with him. I knew God saw my heart's desire to be reunited with both my boys, so I just let Him work.

I know my prayers were heard and had several prophets tell me I would hear from him, but sometimes you feel like you hang on to a thin thread. However, I did hold on to what the Lord promised. Then one day about two years ago, after 60 years of not hearing my little boy's voice, Kenneth called me. You can only imagine how I felt. It was one of the happiest days of my life. God had honored my prayer. I was humbled beyond belief. I really am at a loss of words to describe the joy that has been in my heart to be in contact with both my boys after a lifetime of not being with them. To date I have not had the privilege to meet Kenneth face to face, but we talk on the phone and he tells me that he will come this way and see me one day. I pray that day comes quickly because I am so lonesome to see his face.

You know when you walk with the Lord and live a life totally trusting His will for your life, it is a life of peace and joy most of the time. There are those times, however, that you may wonder how long it's going to take Him to work out a prayer request. For me it was about 45 years to see Steve and 60 years to be able to hear Kenneth's voice, but it has been worth the waiting on the Lord to have my deepest heart's desire come to pass. All I can say is that Father God is truly faithful!

BUILDING RELATIONSHIP

I HAVE SHARED WITH YOU MY LIFE up to date. I would like to share now some of the personal lessons I have learned about relationship with the Lord.

Yes, I believe that life is a journey. Each new day brings with it an expectancy of something wonderful in God. I would like to share a couple of my personal experiences I have had on my journey to explain why I feel the faithfulness of our loving creator is worth everything we go through in this life. I wish I could say that I have always been God's little sweet darling, but as you have read my life story you can see that I battled depression, grief, heartache, rebellion against God, and on another note also love, joy, peace and contentment. I must say contentment is the greatest of all attributes that I am very grateful to have been able to accomplish with the help of the Lord. All the valleys and mountains have taught me exactly who my Father is. I've had to learn to allow the Holy Spirit to work in my life and teach me how to become a child of God.

Not everyone understands the processes we go through as children of God. The Scriptures tell us that He will rebuke and chasten those He loves. I know I am loved greatly because of the things He has done in my life. People say they can't wait to get to heaven to meet the Lord. I have to say that I have met the Lord and the relationship we have is what will take me to my eternal home.

The experiences I have gone through are what has built my faith to learn to trust the Lord. Were they rough you may ask and I would answer, "Well they weren't a piece of cake!" Read for yourself and hopefully you will understand how the love of God will work in you and bring you to the place of relationship with Him that He desires.

OVERCOMING PREJUDICES:

One morning I got up, and I was very ill. I thought I had pneumonia. I had never been this sick since I battled cancer, but I knew something was wrong. Ruth and Frank had gone on a trip to Georgia and I had stayed at home to take care of things, so I was alone. I prayed and prayed for God to heal me, but nothing happened except my getting worse. It was like a tug of war inside me. I had always trusted God for healing, and He had never failed to answer my prayer for healing. Needless to say I got serious about my prayer for healing. I ask God to show me if I had anything in my life that was displeasing to Him. I was very sincere about this request. It was not a fly by night prayer. I knew I was very ill.

As I sat in my prayer room meditating on the Lord, all at once a sheet appeared on the wall in front of me. On the sheet were written the words prejudice, judgmental attitude, pride, and self-righteousness. I was so humbled by my vision and even more so as the Spirit began to show me how each one of these wrong attributes had been in my heart.

I was prideful because I had received such a great healing when I was healed of cancer. The truth is that it was just a tool

God used to show me how merciful and how much He loved me. It wasn't meant to kill me but to heal me from my broken life. Oh don't think it would not have killed me if I had chosen to walk away instead of toward God, but it was His mercy that gave me that choice. Because I chose to give my life to Jesus, I was healed both physically and spiritually.

I am not saying that cancer is the same tool for everybody. Each individual has their own set of circumstances and trials to go through. I only know that to me cancer represented graveyard death, and Jesus offered me life if I would choose Him at that critical time of my life. I will forever, and I mean forever, be grateful I made that choice. I believe Father God gives that same choice to every person. Jesus represents the choice for life, and whether or not it gives us physical life or not, it will always give us eternal life by saying yes to Him.

What I did not realize when I became sick was that I had let my conversion and salvation from cancer make me prideful. I had become self-righteous, prejudice, and very judgmental of people who went to doctors. I had had great victory up to that point in receiving healing for any ailment I had. But God was determined to show me how I had missed the mark of being a true Christian and had gotten cold and indifferent towards people who suffered illness.

Having religion leaves us without compassion. Having Christianity makes us like Christ and He is compassion. Not to justify sin or make allowances for wrong but to realize that anyone can become ensnared in a fault or have a weakness that will cause them to drift in the wrong direction. We who are spiritual are supposed to restore these in love back into God's grace.

As I cried and prayed, the Lord spoke to me and told me to go to the doctor. I did argue for a moment with Him by expressing the fact that I had always trusted Him for healing but His answer was loud and clear. He told me to go because I would learn not to condemn others who needed doctors and chose to go.

When Ruth came home and found me ill, she took me to the doctor. He told me that I had Thyroid Disease and would have been dead in two weeks if I had not came in for diagnosis and treatment. I was stunned to say the least. Again I had to face life or death. I did not realize that I had sin in my life. I thought I was doing all I knew to do to walk with the Lord.

I think of how easily I could have died from my Thyroid problem and if I had to face the Father God with all that sin in my life I would not have made it to Heaven. The only thing that saved me was His compassion and love for me. He knew that I truly loved Him and I asked for Him to show me if there was anything in me that He was not pleased with. He was faithful to do that and allow me forgiveness, and through the doctor He gave me healing.

Some people think once they accept Jesus into their heart that from that point on it is all taken care of. Not true at all. Accepting Jesus and confessing past sins is the first step of spiritual healing. From that point on we must stay humble before God and always be open to the Holy Spirit. Living the Christian life, or Christ centered life, is a daily soul searching and submission to a Loving God who wants us walk uprightly before Him. That is the only way we truly become the light of the World. Letting Christ be formed in us is more that words and that was a lesson I never want to forget.

SUBMISSION TO GOD'S WILL:

Again in 2012 I faced some pretty dramatic health issues. I was having some weak spells and they seemed to be getting worse. After several trips to the doctor and emergency room, the doctors decided I had pneumonia. I spent the night in the hospital and after going home on medication I still had the same symptoms. I finally ended up in the hospital for 6 days with pneumonia.

While in the hospital they did an MRI on my lungs. Little did I know how dangerous that was for someone with a pace maker. I would soon find out though. When I finally got to go home I could not seem to get my strength back. I still suffered with shortness of breath and other symptoms. I ended up in the emergency room in another town where my heart doctor had an office. The ER doctor referred me to him for follow up. After checking my pace maker they decided it was not working properly. The wires had been burned during the MRI and needed to be replaced.

That procedure was fairly simple and only required an overnight hospital stay. Unfortunately, my symptoms did not go away. I was continuing to have dizzy spells and shortness of breath. My heart doctor decided that a test was necessary to look for heart blockages. After the test it was confirmed that I needed stints in some of the arteries. They put three stints in and after a night in the hospital I got to go home.

It took a couple of weeks to gain my strength back. Needless to say during that time I did a lot of soul searching. It's not that I am not ready to go home to be with the Lord, but I have some unfinished promises He has given me, and I want to see them come to pass before I leave this world.

My experience with the Lord is that if I sincerely desire an answer about something and am willing to fast and pray about it, He will show me what is going on. I am very grateful for that. So, I sought and He showed!

You know they always use the phrase; "behind the scenes". Well there were circumstances going on behind the scenes of my health issues.

For some time God had been dealing with me about giving up some of my obligations that were draining my time and strength. I had been church secretary for over 20 years and still had the full time job of Granny's Cottages. I also was what you might say the general gopher for the pastor. I ran all the errands associated with events planned for the church. None of the things I did were wrong or bad, but the thing that got me into trouble with the Lord is that I ignored Him about slowing down and letting someone else take some of the responsibilities. In a church of about 300 people there are plenty of people capable and willing to do some of the jobs I did for the pastor.

A pastor is like any other leader of an organization. They have to have loyal trustworthy people to handle the leadership jobs. I am very close to my pastor and his wife being willing to serve in any way I can, fell into being the main person to carry the entire load. It was years in the making actually. I have been with this pastor for over 20 years, and he trusts me completely. As the years went by, I just took over helping him with the running of church business. It was not planned but became a way of life for both of us. I know that God was not upset about me serving in the church, but it was just time to allow someone else to start carrying the load. At 83 God was saying I want you to slow down and quit wearing yourself out carrying a load that so many others can do. When the church was small planning luncheons and outings, doing the bookkeeping, planning for incoming speakers, etc. was very easy, but for a large congregation it takes more than one hat to accomplish the job.

I wish I could say that past experience of ignoring the voice of God taught me to never do it again, but in fact, we seem to forget from one lesson to another. I think I felt like I was the only one that could do the jobs for the church. Perhaps it was just habit. I didn't want to disappoint my pastor, and maybe I enjoyed being needed or the feeling of importance, I'm not really sure. All I know is that my failure to listen when the Holy Spirit began dealing with me caused God to chasten me.

I know religious people may disagree with me and say to me that God does not allow sickness to happen to His children. I believe that my own disobedience caused God to withdraw His protection, and because of my own stubbornness, I fell prey to sickness.

The Bible records incidents when people would ask Jesus why were people sick or demon possessed. He gave many different reasons. I like to relate to the story He told the crowd in John chapter 11 that the sickness was imposed for the glory of God. I know what I went through was to bring glory to God not only for me but for those who would receive my testimony.

I had actually become rebellious to the will of God for my life. I'm not proud of that, but the truth is the truth. I simply refused to listen when the Holy Spirit dealt with me about my life. I was quick to tell others about obeying the Lord,, and I didn't listen myself. I would even get mad when people would say something to me about slowing down. It pricked my heart because I knew it was truth. When we act this way with God we leave Him no option but to deal with us in the manner He sees fit. With me it was through my health. With others it may be finances, children, houses, lands, jobs, etc........ Believe me He knows what our weaknesses are and how to get our attention.

People may just brush something off as an attack of the devil or coincidence when something happens, but I can't find anywhere in the Bible where God leaves the well being of His children up to coincidence. He has angels watching over us, the Holy Spirit living in us, and Jesus is always there to lead us. We really don't have an excuse for not knowing the will of God except we just don't seek Him for it or we ignore what He tell us because it doesn't agree with what we want.

I wonder how many wonderful things I have missed or you have missed simply because we refused to listen when the Spirit spoke to us. We settle into comfortable life styles or places and we don't want to change anything, so we turn off any instruction that might be different than what we have planned for our lives. When God deals with us about change it may just be a changing of our mind sets or a change of life style but whatever it is, if we will listen, it will keep us in His perfect will. This is the peace of God that He desires for us.

WHAT'S AHEAD?

I DON'T THINK ANY ONE OF US can predict all that is ahead of us in God on this earth, but the promises He has given me of many more adventures I know I can count on coming to pass.

I have been prophesied to many times that I will travel to Africa. I look forward to that. I want to see what God is doing over there to help those people. From all I have seen, He is really moving and saving those people. I look forward to that trip.

I also look forward to meeting in person, after 60 years, my oldest son Kenneth and his wife. Also getting to meet my grandchildren for the first time is almost more excitement that I can contain. I love them already and can't wait to give each one a hug. I also look forward to seeing my youngest son, Steve, again.

These are my personal promises that God has assured me will come to pass before He takes me home. As for all the promises He has given us in His word, I have those to count on too.

Life truly is a journey. Sometimes we make our journey more difficult by our own self will and desires, and sometimes we have to just wait on God to work out the details so He can bring a promise to pass. I found a key to receiving those promises fulfilled and that key is submission and obedience to the Spirit of God. Sometimes His will for us goes against everything we want or desire, but if we allow Him to take over our life with His plan for us we can find a place of peace and rest.

My life started in a little country house in Vermont. My childhood was one of pain. By running away at the age of 12, I had to grow up way too fast. Because of that, I made some very bad choices which over and over changed the course of my life until one day the Lord put my life in the balance with cancer. He made Himself very real to me through that journey. Just as He did Abraham, He led me into a strange country that would become my home for the rest of my earthly life. He has given me a land of milk and honey, and that Abraham, was not without test and trials. Now at age 84, I am seeing my seed promise come to pass. I truly can say I can testify to Psalm 23 as a beacon of my life. It really says it all for me!

Psalm 23

> "The Lord is my Shepherd; I shall not want. He maketh me to lie down in green pastures: He leadeth me beside the still waters. He restoreth my soul: He leadeth me in the paths of righteousness for His name's sake. Yea, though I walk through the valley of the shadow of death, I will fear no evil: for thou art with me; thy rod and thy staff they comfort me. Thou preparest a table before me in the presence of mine enemies: Thou anointest my head with oil; my cup runneth over. Surely goodness and mercy shall follow me all the days of my life; and I will dwell in the house of the Lord forever." KJV

www.ingramcontent.com/pod-product-compliance
Lightning Source LLC
Chambersburg PA
CBHW020408290526
45785CB00005B/2469